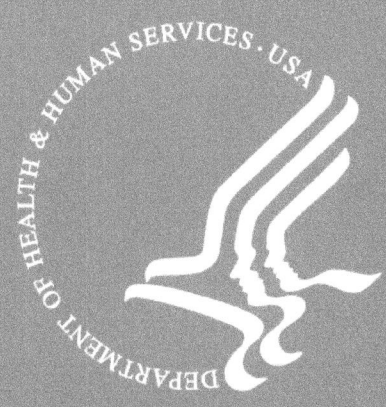

U.S. Department of Health & Human Services

2010 National Vaccine Plan

Protecting the Nation's Health through Immunization

U.S. Department of Health & Human Services

2010 National Vaccine Plan

Protecting the Nation's Health through Immunization

Table of Contents

---

1. Please note that the Appendices can be found on the National Vaccine Plan website at www.hhs.gov/nvpo/vacc_plan/index. As the Plan is a "living document," the Appendices will be updated on an ongoing basis.

Acronyms and Abbreviations

ACA	Affordable Care Act (comprised of the Patient Protection and Affordable Care Act and the Health Care and Education Reconciliation Act of 2010)	IHS	Indian Health Service
		IIS	Immunization Information Systems
		IOM	Institute of Medicine
ACF	Administration for Children and Families	NGO	Non-Governmental Organization
		NIH	National Institutes of Health
ACIP	Advisory Committee on Immunization Practices	NVAC	National Vaccine Advisory Committee
AEFI	Adverse Event Following Immunization	NVP	National Vaccine Program
		NVPO	National Vaccine Program Office
AIDS	Acquired Immune Deficiency Syndrome	ONC	Office of the National Coordinator for Health Information Technology
AHRQ	Agency for Healthcare Research and Quality	P.L.	Public Law
		TB	Tuberculosis
ASPR	Assistant Secretary for Preparedness and Response	UNICEF	United Nation's Children's Fund (formerly United Nations International Children's Emergency Fund)
BARDA	Biomedical Advanced Research and Development Authority		
CDC	Centers for Disease Control and Prevention	USAID	U.S. Agency for International Development
CICP	Countermeasures Injury Compensation Program	VA	Department of Veterans Affairs
		VICP	National Vaccine Injury Compensation Program
CMS	Centers for Medicare and Medicaid Services	VPD	Vaccine-Preventable Disease
DoD	Department of Defense	WHO	World Health Organization
DHS	Department of Homeland Security		
DoJ	Department of Justice		
EHR	Electronic Health Records		
FDA	Food and Drug Administration		
GAVI	Global Alliance for Vaccines and Immunizations		
GHI	Global Health Initiative		
HBV	Hepatitis B Virus		
HHS	U.S. Department of Health and Human Services		
Hib	*Haemophilus influenzae* type b		
HIV	Human Immunodeficiency Virus		
HP	Healthy People		
HPV	Human papillomavirus		
HRSA	Health Resources and Services Administration		

"To raise new questions, new possibilities, to regard old problems from a new angle, requires creative imagination and marks real advance in science."

- **Albert Einstein**

Executive Summary

The 20th century could be considered the century of vaccines. The life spans of Americans increased by more than thirty years in large part because of vaccines, and mortality from infectious diseases in the United States decreased 14-fold.[2] Death or disability from many once-common diseases is now rare in the U.S. A child born in the U.S. today can now be protected against 17 serious diseases and conditions through immunization. The widespread use of vaccines has helped to eradicate smallpox worldwide and eliminate polio, measles and rubella in the U.S. Globally, vaccination saves 2 to 3 million lives per year.[3]

Vaccines have the unique quality of protecting both individuals and communities. However, they have been so effective for many years in preventing and eliminating a number of serious infectious diseases that the significant contributions that vaccines make to our society and its health may have faded from public consciousness. Before the development and widespread use of safe and effective vaccines, infectious diseases threatened the lives of millions of children and adults in this country and abroad. What were once referred to as the common diseases of childhood are now vaccine-preventable diseases (VPDs). In the U.S., children are no longer crippled cases by polio nor killed by infections such as diphtheria or *Haemophilus influenzae* type B (Hib). Vaccines also help prevent cancers caused by human papillomavirus (HPV) and hepatitis B virus (HBV).

The 2010 National Vaccine Plan provides a vision for the U.S. vaccine and immunization enterprise for the next decade. The Plan articulates a comprehensive strategy to enhance all aspects of vaccines and vaccination including: research and development, supply, financing, distribution, safety, informed decision making by consumers and health care providers, VPD surveillance, vaccine effectiveness and use monitoring, and global cooperation. The actions contained in the strategies of the Plan are conditional and are subject to the availability of resources.

The scope of the Plan is broad and addresses vaccines and key vaccine-related issues for the U.S. and its global partners. It provides a strategic approach for preventing infectious diseases and improving the public's health through vaccination for the coming decade. Although vaccines are being developed to treat diseases and conditions (therapeutic vaccines) and for non-infectious diseases, the focus of this Plan is on vaccines for the prevention of infectious diseases as guided by the law that established the National Vaccine Program (NVP).[4]

2. American Academy of Pediatrics. Prologue. In: Pickering LK, ed. Red Book: 2009 Report of the Committee on Infectious Diseases. 28th ed. Elk Grove Village, IL: American Academy of Pediatrics; 2009:1-2.

3. World Health Organization and United Nations Children's Fund. Global Immunization Vision and Strategy, 2006--2015. Geneva, Switzerland: World Health Organization and United Nations Children's Fund; 2005. Available at www.who.int/vaccines/GIVS/english/GIVS_Final_17Oct05.pdf.

4. Public Law (P.L.) 99-660 established the National Vaccine Program, and required the National Vaccine Program to focus on prevention of infectious diseases and adverse reactions to vaccines.

The Plan has five broad goals:

Goal 1:
Develop new and improved vaccines.

Goal 2:
Enhance the vaccine safety system.

Goal 3:
Support communications to enhance informed vaccine decision-making.

Goal 4:
Ensure a stable supply of, access to, and better use of recommended vaccines in the United States.

Goal 5:
Increase global prevention of death and disease through safe and effective vaccination.

Existing national and global vaccine-related initiatives, such as improvements in regulatory science, the development of medical countermeasures for emergencies, and global health partnerships are embedded within the Plan. Strategies of this Plan will also be coordinated with those developed through other federal efforts. One example is the National Prevention, Health Promotion and Public Health Council, established in the 2010 Affordable Care Act (ACA). The Council will coordinate federal prevention, wellness, and public health activities, and develop a national strategy to improve the nation's health.

In conjunction with other federal efforts like the National Prevention and Health Promotion Strategy, Healthy People (HP) 2020, and the Public Health Emergency Medical Countermeasures Enterprise Review, the 2010 National Vaccine Plan provides the strategic guidance to build a stronger preventive health system. It will help bridge disparities in use of, and access to vaccines, and will provide innovative strategies to guide the nation's vaccine enterprise across the next decade and beyond.

Purpose and Background

The purpose of the 2010 National Vaccine Plan is to provide strategic direction for the coordination of the vaccine and immunization enterprise for the NVP. The Program's goals are to prevent infectious diseases and their sequelae and reduce adverse reactions to vaccines in the U.S. The Plan will achieve this through coordinated implementation of a strategic vision implemented by vaccine and immunization stakeholders across and outside of the federal government.

Background

Federal involvement in vaccination programs targeting civilian and military populations has a rich history that includes research and development, assuring safety and effectiveness, supporting delivery, and developing mechanisms for reporting adverse events following immunization. Recognizing the need for increased coordination of these activities, the NVP was established by Congress in 1986.[5] Congress called for the development of a National Vaccine Plan to guide activities in pursuit of program goals. The initial Plan, completed in 1994, defined activities to achieve the program's mission through coordinated action by federal agencies, state and local governments, and private sector partners including manufacturers and health care providers.

The nation's vaccine enterprise has made considerable progress since the first National Vaccine Plan. Through routine vaccination, a child born today can be protected against 17 diseases and conditions while one born in 1995 could be protected against only nine. Growing scientific knowledge coupled with advances in biotechnology provides possibilities for new and improved vaccines. Many of the financial barriers that once limited widespread use of vaccines have been overcome. A myriad of enhanced tools are available for communicating accurate information about vaccines and for ensuring that vaccines are safe and effective. A broad range of public and private stakeholders have become essential to the vaccine enterprise.

Ironically, the public health victory witnessed from the use of vaccines has created a public health challenge: because vaccines have reduced the impact and awareness of many infectious diseases, some have begun to question the value and need for vaccines. In addition, the long-term effects (e.g., cancer) of some VPDs (e.g., HBV and HPV) may not be visible to the public, thus diminishing the perceived value of vaccination. Thus, this Plan comes at a critical time for this nation and its health as it engages on these issues and as there is an increased focus on the importance of preventive health for the U.S. and its citizens.

---

5. P.L. 99-660

Mission, Perspective, and Scope

The 2010 National Vaccine Plan provides a strategic approach for preventing infectious diseases and improving the public's health through vaccination.

The scope of the Plan is broad, including vaccines and vaccine-related issues for the U.S. and global communities. As guided by the statute that established the NVP, the focus for this Plan is prevention of infectious diseases and adverse reactions to vaccines.[6] The Plan incorporates current initiatives, such as the long recognized need to develop vaccines against human immunodeficiency virus/acquired immune deficiency syndrome (HIV/AIDS), tuberculosis (TB), and malaria, and programs to enhance medical countermeasures, regulatory science, and vaccine production. A ten-year horizon was set for the Plan to align with HP 2020 goals (see Appendix 1 for more details[7]).

2010 National Vaccine Plan Structure

The 2010 National Vaccine Plan provides a comprehensive approach to reduce infectious diseases and their sequelae and reduce adverse reactions to vaccines through coordinated efforts of federal, state, local, multinational and non-governmental stakeholders. Recognizing that success is facilitated by careful planning that includes defining specific activities, milestones and measurable outcomes, an implementation plan will be developed based on this plan and released in 2011. With a ten-year horizon, this framework recognizes and anticipates that emerging science, new opportunities, and changing circumstances will guide the course of the Plan. Annual monitoring of progress and a mid-course review will promote both accountability and flexibility.

The Plan is built around five broad goals:

Goal 1:
Develop new and improved vaccines.

Goal 2:
Enhance the vaccine safety system.

Goal 3:
Support communications to enhance informed vaccine decision-making.

Goal 4:
Ensure a stable supply of, access to, and better use of recommended vaccines in the United States.

Goal 5:
Increase global prevention of death and disease through safe and effective vaccination.

Each goal is supported by objectives that will be pursued through a defined set of strategies. Reaching goals and objectives generally requires action by many stakeholders in the vaccine and immunization enterprise. The Implementation Plan, to be written during 2011, will describe the action steps and measurable indicators for key Plan objectives and strategies.

---

6. P.L. 99-660

7. Please note that the Appendices can be found on the National Vaccine Plan website at www.hhs.gov/nvpo/vacc_ plan/index. As the Plan is a "living document," the Appendices will be updated on an ongoing basis.

Progress Since the 1994 Plan

The 2010 National Vaccine Plan builds on the many achievements of the vaccine and immunization enterprise prior to and since the establishment of the NVP in 1986 and the completion of the first National Vaccine Plan in 1994. New vaccines have been licensed to expand the number of infections that can be prevented, and more effectively and safely prevent some diseases for which earlier generation vaccines already existed. In addition, federal immunization financing programs have reduced or eliminated many financial barriers to vaccination, particularly for children. The number of infections caused by VPDs has decreased significantly while vaccination coverage in the U.S. has increased, and coverage for many vaccines has reached record levels. More robust systems have been developed to identify adverse events following immunization and to assess potential associations of those events with vaccination. Globally, the U.S. has worked with multilateral and bilateral partners and non-governmental organizations (NGOs) in contributing to improvements in child health status and the prevention of hundreds of thousands of child deaths each year through improved vaccine coverage and introduction of new vaccines. Of the fourteen anticipated outcomes included in the 1994 National Vaccine Plan, most were substantially or fully achieved (see Appendix 2).

Unfortunately, many of the challenges that stimulated establishment of the NVP and the development of the 1994 National Vaccine Plan remain relevant today. Vaccine shortages and interruptions have occurred for many routinely recommended vaccines. Despite improved vaccination coverage among children, recent VPD outbreaks in the U.S. serve as reminders that these diseases still occur. Among older adults both vaccination coverage and the effectiveness of some routinely recommended vaccines remain sub-optimal. Disparities exist in adult vaccination rates between racial and ethnic groups. As the cost of vaccination has increased, financial barriers to vaccination have emerged for health departments, health care providers, and the public. Significant scientific challenges remain in the development of safe and effective vaccines against existing global health threats, such as HIV, TB and malaria. Vaccines that have been developed and are in use in industrialized countries have the potential to make major contributions to health in developing countries, but are currently underused in many places. Additionally, emerging infections and the persistent threat of natural and intentional infectious disease pose new challenges for vaccine development and regulation, manufacturing, vaccine delivery and access in the U.S. and abroad.

U.S. Immunization Framework

Disease prevention and enhanced vaccine safety are ultimate outcomes of a successful vaccination program. Identifying objectives and strategies that lead to and sustain these outcomes is facilitated by understanding the many processes or determinants of these outcomes.

To protect individuals and communities from VPDs, vaccines must be administered to the public. Vaccination begins with the identification of public health priorities, which are informed by disease surveillance data and information on the public health burden of the diseases that vaccines can effectively and safely prevent. Vaccine research and licensure follows. After the licensure of a vaccine and the Advisory Committee on Immunization Practices (ACIP) and medical organizations' recommendation for its use, a vaccine must be distributed, stored, and handled appropriately. Vaccine payment and reimbursement policies are important for ensuring receipt and use of the vaccine. Communications and public and provider outreach help support informed decision-making about vaccination. Attitudes, vaccination coverage and the effectiveness of disease prevention also are influenced by issues related to vaccine safety and effectiveness.

Development of the 2010 National Vaccine Plan

The 2010 National Vaccine Plan, under the coordination of the U.S. Department of Health and Human Services (HHS) National Vaccine Program Office (NVPO), is the product of deliberation, analysis, and input from multiple federal agencies, and it incorporates broad public and stakeholder input. NVPO is the principal coordinating office for the NVP and is responsible for providing leadership, facilitating coordination, and monitoring progress of the 2010 National Vaccine Plan during implementation.

Relevant federal government agencies (see Appendix 3) identified key objectives and strategies as pathways to success for each of the five goals. NVPO consulted with the National Vaccine Advisory Committee (NVAC), federal agencies, domestic and international stakeholders, and the public regularly about the development of the Plan. A national stakeholder meeting was convened to discuss the first draft of the Plan. In addition to the national stakeholder meeting, NVPO obtained input through several mechanisms:

- Comments gathered by an Institute of Medicine (IOM) committee[8] at five public meetings that focused on the different goals in the Plan;

- The IOM committee's final report;[9]

- Input from federal vaccine advisory committee members;

- Meetings with domestic and international stakeholders; and

- Input from the public in three public meetings and through public comment in response to a notice in the Federal Register.

Additional information about the development of the National Vaccine Plan is available at *www.hhs.gov/nvpo/vacc_plan/index.*

Coordination with Other Federal Initiatives

The 2010 National Vaccine Plan will support relevant strategic health priorities and key interagency collaborations for the nation issued by the Secretary of HHS, which include the following: to promote early childhood health and development, to accelerate the process of scientific discovery to improve patient care, and to improve global health.[10] Global health plays an important role in the national security of the U.S. population and populations worldwide, and as such the Plan is of import to all agencies involved in global health activities, including the Department of State and the U.S. Agency for International Development (USAID). U.S. involvement in global vaccine issues can reduce worldwide transmission of VPDs, strengthen health systems, and foster bilateral and international partnerships.

In addition, the 2010 National Vaccine Plan has direct relevance to the goals of the ACA, the comprehensive health care reform law enacted in March 2010, which expands access to preventive care, including vaccines, by requiring health plans to cover preventive services without charging a deductible, copayment, or coinsurance. Individuals enrolled in these new group or individual health plans will have access to the vaccines recommended by the ACIP prior to

---

8. HHS requested the formation of an IOM committee specifically to gather public input and provide recommendations on priorities for the 2010 National Vaccine Plan.

9. Available at www.iom.edu/Reports/2009/Priorities-for-the-National-Vaccine-Plan.

10. U.S. Department of Health and Human Services. Secretary's Strategic Initiatives & Key Inter-Agency Collaborations. Available at www.hhs.gov/secretary/about/priorities.

September 2009 with no co-payments or other cost-sharing requirements when those services are delivered by an in-network provider. These new health plans will be required to cover new ACIP recommendations made after September 2009 without cost-sharing in the next plan year that occurs one year after the date of the recommendation. In addition to expanding access to immunization under the preventive services rules, the ACA includes the following immunization-related provisions:

• Provides authority to states to purchase adult vaccines with state funds from federally-negotiated contracts.

• Reauthorizes the Section 317 Immunization Grant Program, which makes available federally purchased vaccines and grants to all 50 states, the District of Columbia, five large urban areas, and territories and protectorates to provide immunization services to priority populations.

• Requires a General Accountability Office study and report to Congress about Medicare beneficiary access to recommended vaccines under the Medicare Part D benefit.

More information about the new preventive services requirements can be found at: *www.healthcare.gov/center/regulations/prevention/recommendations.*

Strategies identified in the Plan will be coordinated with those in the National Health Security Strategy, the Global Health Initiative (GHI), the National Strategy for Pandemic Influenza, and other national strategic plans that relate to immunization and vaccines. In particular, this work will be coordinated with the National Prevention, Health Promotion and Public Health Council's priorities, which will integrate federal prevention, wellness, and public health activities, and develop the National Prevention and Health Promotion Strategy to improve the nation's health. All of these efforts will complement the National Strategy for Quality Improvement in Health Care, also described in the ACA.

The Plan aligns with quality of care improvement initiatives under the Children's Health Insurance Program Reauthorization Act and complements the Centers for Medicare and Medicaid (CMS)'s work to improve access to and measurement of mandatory health care services delivered children enrolled in Medicaid through the Early and Periodic Screening, Diagnostic, and Treatment Program. The Plan also supports the GHI, which focuses on improving the health of women, newborns, and children worldwide through strengthened health systems and through coordinated, results-oriented, country-led approaches. Additionally, the Plan complements other initiatives including the U.S. President's Emergency Plan For AIDS Relief, which assists countries in strengthening their health systems and providing comprehensive prevention, care, and treatment to combat the global epidemic of HIV/AIDS and diplomatic efforts to build global partnerships in preparation for pandemic influenza and other pandemic diseases. For a full list of relevant plans please see Appendix 4.

Understanding the extensive scope of the vaccine and immunization enterprise, the Plan also encompasses relevant strategic visions within other federal agencies. These include the HP 2020 objectives as well as the full spectrum of strategies articulated in the effort to develop medical countermeasures against bioterrorist threats, the threat of pandemics, and new and emerging infectious disease threats.[11]

---

11. For example, see BARDA strategic plan at www.hhs.gov/aspr/barda/phemce/enterprise/strategy/index.

Implementation Opportunities and Challenges

Many factors may affect achievement of the 2010 National Vaccine Plan. Opportunities may emerge that facilitate rapid progress and achievement of objectives sooner than anticipated. Scientific, technological, health care financing, or communications advances also could emerge, enabling rapid achievement of the vision laid forth by the Plan, superseding its objectives and goals. Conversely, existing challenges and barriers may be more difficult to overcome than anticipated and new challenges may surface.

The 2010 National Vaccine Plan will rely on sound science and includes measurable goals, timelines, and accountability measures for the elements that have been identified as highest priority as noted in Table 1. These priorities take into account the suggestions of the IOM, the NVAC, and the agencies involved in developing, implementing and evaluating the 2010 National Vaccine Plan. These priorities also provide strategic action steps to ensure that the nation has a robust immunization program; they are not however intended to be a comprehensive list of all activities related to vaccines and immunizations. The actions described in the Plan are conditional, serve as a guideline for future development, and are subject to the availability of resources.

Indicators for tracking progress in meeting each of these priorities are under development and will be included in an Implementation Plan to be released in 2011. These indicators will represent the federal government's plan for measuring progress toward meeting the Plan's goals and include immediate, short-term, and longer-term actions. In 2011, NVPO will consult with federal agencies to implement these priorities and develop indicators for 2012 and beyond and update them as necessary. Additionally, as federal agencies begin to implement the Plan and as discussions continue with stakeholders, new indicators may also be developed.

Implementing the 2010 National Vaccine Plan does not fall to the federal government alone. The success of this plan will require states, tribal and local governments, components of the health care delivery system, communities and other stakeholders to work together to ensure a coordinated and comprehensive immunization program. See Appendix 5 for a list of immunization stakeholders. The priorities and the Plan are intended to serve as a catalyst for all stakeholders to develop their own implementation plans for achieving the goals of the 2010 National Vaccine Plan.

Table 1:

National Vaccine Plan Priorities for Implementation

A.	Develop a catalogue of priority vaccine targets of domestic and global health importance (**Goal 1**).
B.	Strengthen the science base for the development and licensure of new vaccines (**Goals 1 and 2**).
C.	Enhance timely detection and verification of vaccine safety signals and develop a vaccine safety scientific agenda (**Goal 2**).
D.	Increase awareness of vaccines, vaccine-preventable diseases, and the benefits/risks of immunization among the public, providers, and other stakeholders (**Goal 3**).
E.	Use evidence-based science to enhance vaccine-preventable disease surveillance, measurement of vaccine coverage, and measurement of vaccine effectiveness (**Goal 4**).
F.	Eliminate financial barriers for providers and consumers to facilitate access to routinely recommended vaccines (**Goal 4**).
G.	Create an adequate and stable supply of routinely recommended vaccines and vaccines for public health preparedness (**Goal 4**).
H.	Increase and improve the use of interoperable health information technology and electronic health records (**Goal 4**).
I.	Improve global surveillance for vaccine-preventable diseases and strengthen global health information systems to monitor vaccine coverage, effectiveness, and safety (**Goal 5**).
J.	Support global introduction and availability of new and under-utilized vaccines to prevent diseases of public health importance (**Goal 5**).

Goal 1:
Develop new and improved vaccines

Introduction
The greatest and most rapid changes in health occurred during the last century, primarily attributed to a higher standard of living, improved public health measures, and the application of science-based medicine. In addition to clean water, sanitation, and the use of antibiotics, vaccines are an essential part of these public health achievements. Vaccine research and development as well as the implementation of effective vaccine delivery programs has led to the eradication and elimination of several once-common serious infectious diseases.

Discovery begins with the recognition of an infectious disease burden and the opportunity to prevent it through immunization. Basic scientific research brings ideas forward into the product development pathway toward the ultimate goal of translating these ideas into safe and effective medical products. Safety and efficacy testing are conducted at every step of this product development pathway. Both basic and targeted research is the basis for the development of vaccine candidates and new vaccine platforms that offer greater flexibility in vaccine development and production. New tools, such as efficient antigen identification techniques, coupled with a profoundly greater understanding of the immune response are available to define basic mechanisms of disease to support design and development of novel and improved vaccines. Determining "proof of concept" regarding immunogenicity and safety follows – initially in pre-clinical studies in animals and then in humans to further evaluate safety and efficacy. Finally, researchers conduct scientific characterization of the vaccine and the process for producing it, including scaling the manufacturing process to commercial levels before vaccines are moved into human testing.

Vaccines are developed through public-private partnerships – including researchers, government, manufacturers, purchasers, and policy-makers – who have been successful at bringing new vaccines to licensure for broad use. These partnerships are central to the success of vaccine innovations. Through targeted investments in science and technology, such partnerships have led to the development of hundreds of vaccine candidates at various stages of maturity in the development pipeline. The Global HIV Enterprise is an example of unprecedented collaboration among organizations worldwide, including the National Institutes of Health (NIH), the International AIDS Vaccine Initiative, USAID, the Bill and Melinda Gates Foundation, and many others working together to accelerate the development of a preventive HIV vaccine.

Because vaccine development is time- and resource-intensive, establishing and understanding priorities for development and encouraging collaboration between stakeholders is essential in addressing the challenges of developing new and improved vaccines. Fostering continued investment from all sectors is critical as technological approaches and disease threats expand amid increasing costs to develop, license, and deliver vaccines.

The aim of Goal 1 is to develop new and improved vaccines and to address the upstream research and development aspects of vaccines for domestic and global health priorities. The research needs of other aspects of the vaccine enterprise (e.g., program implementation, distribution logistics, communication) are included within other goals in the Plan.

Objectives

Objective 1.1
Prioritize new vaccine targets of domestic and global public health importance.

Strategies:
1.1.1
Develop and implement a process for prioritizing and evaluating new vaccine targets of domestic and global public health importance. This catalogue of vaccine targets (including improved vaccines) should include an analysis of barriers to development.

1.1.2
Conduct and improve disease surveillance of existing pathogens and optimize methods to detect new pathogens to continuously inform the priorities for potential new vaccines.

Objective 1.2
Support research to develop and manufacture new vaccine candidates and improve current vaccines to prevent infectious diseases.

Strategies:
1.2.1
Conduct and support expanded vaccine research to meet medical and public health needs. Establish surveillance systems or studies to better assess disease burden in specific target populations including neonates, infants, children, older adults, pregnant women, immunocompromised individuals, and other at-risk individuals.

1.2.2
Advance research and development toward new and/or improved vaccines that prevent infectious diseases and their sequelae, including those that protect against emerging, re-emerging, and important biodefense-related pathogens.

1.2.3
Advance the science of neonatal and maternal immunity including immunization and the development of immunological models to study maternal immunization and effects on offspring.

1.2.4
Develop a process that identifies current vaccines that would benefit from improved performance characteristics (e.g., effectiveness, safety, number of doses, stability, and/or vaccine administration characteristics) that can be used in the evaluation and licensure process.

1.2.5
Develop new approaches to vaccine manufacturing (e.g., rapid, flexible, and cost-effective) to meet demands for efficient, expandable vaccine production capacity while also meeting needs related to other public health emergency threats such as international emerging diseases.

Objective 1.3
Support research on novel and improved vaccine delivery methods.

Strategies:
1.3.1
Develop and evaluate new and improved alternate delivery methods of vaccine administration to optimize the protective immune response, safety, effectiveness, and/or efficiency (e.g., number of doses).

1.3.2
Expand knowledge regarding the induction and maintenance of vaccine immune responses via different routes of administration (e.g., mucosal surfaces).

Objective 1.4
Increase understanding of the host immune system.

Strategies
1.4.1
Define the capacity and quality of innate and adaptive human immune response to infections among diverse gender, ethnic, racial, age (childhood, adolescence, and adulthood), and health condition status (e.g., autoimmune compromised individuals) populations in order to advance the understanding of immune protection.

1.4.2
Gain a better understanding of how induction and recall of immune memory may inform the development of vaccines that provide life-long protection.

1.4.3
Support development of immunomodulators including vaccine adjuvants that facilitate the appropriate cell-mediated and antibody responses for protection against pathogens with distinct effector requirements.

1.4.4
Expand knowledge of host-related factors that impact severity of disease and vaccine-induced host immune response, and use this information to inform vaccine development.

1.4.5
Develop a database of gene-expression and immunologic responses to selected currently licensed vaccines with a focus on signals that correlate with mechanism of action, protection, safety, and adverse events. Utilize this compendium to inform development of new candidate vaccines and adjuvants.

1.4.6
Study mucosal immunity following vaccination in order to better understand vaccine mechanisms and to provide new, potentially more relevant, correlates of protection against respiratory, enteric, genital, and urinary pathogens.

Objective 1.5

Support product development, evaluation, and production techniques of vaccine candidates and the scientific tools needed for their evaluation.

Strategies

1.5.1

Support applied research to develop rapid and cost-efficient production, and optimize formulations and stability profiles of currently available vaccines.

1.5.2

Support research on and development of more flexible and agile approaches to product development, manufacturing production techniques including multi-use technologies such as platforms, and quality testing procedures (e.g., potency and safety testing).

1.5.3

Improve access to pilot lot manufacturing facilities that produce clinical grade material for evaluating promising vaccine candidates.

1.5.4

Support translational research that accelerates the development of information that can be used in the evaluation and licensure process.

1.5.5

Establish and strengthen public and private partnerships to address urgent needs in vaccine research and development.

Objective 1.6

Improve the tools, standards, and approaches to assess the safety, efficacy, and quality of vaccines.

Strategies

1.6.1

Improve assay development for characterization of novel cell substrates.

1.6.2

Improve efforts to develop, refine, and validate new biomarkers and correlates of immunity.

1.6.3

Develop and improve methods to better assess vaccine efficacy and safety including assessment of new technologies and development of better animal models.

1.6.4

Improve methods for assessing and evaluating vaccine quality, potency, safety, and effectiveness.

Goal 2:
Enhance the vaccine safety system

Introduction

The U.S. has a robust vaccine safety system. The goal of this system is to identify in a timely manner and minimize the occurrence of adverse events from vaccines. Past successes and challenges offer insights into areas where the existing vaccine safety system can be enhanced. Advances in information technology enhance the ability to conduct active surveillance. Improvements in understanding of immunology and genomics create opportunities to better comprehend the immune response and biological mechanisms important for understanding the safety of vaccines.

Vaccine safety is a key element of any immunization program. The vision of Goal 2 is to specifically address safety-related issues, strengthen the system that monitors the safety of vaccines throughout production and use, and advance the safety profile of vaccines.[12] Specifically, this goal aims to prevent adverse events and fully characterize the safety profile of vaccines in a timely manner.

Vaccine safety science is often challenging because it may require studying very rare outcomes. However, tools have been developed that help detect and quantify exceedingly rare events. Importantly, a vaccine safety monitoring system should have the capacity to distinguish a potential increased risk of a vaccine adverse reaction from an adverse event following immunization[13] that is occurring because of other diseases or exposures. Every day, people suffer from heart attacks, severe headaches and other health problems and some of these will naturally coincide with vaccination. Moreover, as the ability of epidemiology to rule out a very rare event is difficult, new technologies and multi-disciplinary research can help elucidate biological mechanisms and subpopulations at increased risk for adverse events and help address these scientific challenges.

Several important vaccine safety issues are addressed in other goals of the 2010 National Vaccine Plan. For example, Goal 1 addresses vaccine research and development that includes the importance of safety assessments in pre-clinical and clinical vaccine evaluation. Issues related to education, risk communications, behavioral science research, and stakeholder engagement on vaccine safety are included in Goal 3. Because vaccine safety is an important component of every immunization program, whether in the U.S. or globally, it is also featured in Goals 4 and 5.

---

12. Throughout Goal 2, the following terms are frequently used: "signal" and "vaccine adverse reaction." These terms as are defined as:

    Signal: While there are multiple definitions of signals, in this document a signal refers to a concern that a vaccine adverse event could be temporally occurring more often than anticipated based on chance alone (i.e., that the event could be related to the receipt of the vaccine). A signal is not proof of causation; rather it represents the need for further evaluation. Signals may arise from a variety of sources, including from pre-licensure clinical trials, case series, surveillance, clinical experience, the literature, expert committee reviews, the media and/or the public.

    Vaccine adverse reaction is an adverse event caused by a vaccine. Vaccine adverse reactions are defined as minor, such as a sore arm or low grade fever, or can be more severe such as anaphylaxis. Vaccine adverse reactions are dichotomized as local (e.g., sore arm, swelling at site of injection) or systemic (e.g., fever, irritability).

13. *Adverse event following immunization* (AEFI) is an adverse event temporally associated with an immunization that may or may not be causally related to the immunization. The term "vaccine adverse event" is also commonly used to convey the same meaning.

Objectives

Objective 2.1
Ensure a robust vaccine safety scientific system that focuses on high priority areas.

Strategies:
2.1.1
Develop, prioritize, and regularly update a national vaccine safety scientific agenda.

2.1.2
Retain current and recruit additional highly trained vaccine safety scientists and clinicians.

2.1.3
Improve laboratory, epidemiological, and statistical methods used in vaccine safety research.

Objective 2.2
Facilitate the timely integration of advances in manufacturing sciences and regulatory approaches relevant to manufacturing, inspection, and oversight to enhance product quality and patient safety.

Strategies:
2.2.1
Facilitate the enhancement of vaccine manufacturing sciences and quality systems, including production technologies, in-process controls and testing, and identification of best practices in preventive quality systems and oversight.

2.2.2
Develop, implement, and periodically reassess risk-based scientific approaches to identify inspectional priorities and best practices.

2.2.3
Develop new scientific methods for both industry and the Food and Drug Administration (FDA) for product quality testing.

2.2.4
Assure that regulations, guidance documents, policies, and procedures that are relevant to vaccine manufacturing, laboratory testing, and quality control incorporate the most current relevant scientific information to promote and enhance product safety.

Objective 2.3
Enhance timely detection and verification of vaccine safety signals.

Strategies
2.3.1
Improve the effectiveness and timeliness of signal identification and assessment through coordinated use of passive and active surveillance systems, and from providers and the public.

2.3.2
Improve the process for assessing AEFI signals to determine which signals should be evaluated further in epidemiological and clinical studies.

Objective 2.4:

Improve timeliness of the evaluation of vaccine safety signals, especially when 1) a high-priority new vaccine safety concern emerges or 2) when a new vaccine is recommended, vaccination recommendations are expanded, or during public health emergencies such as in an influenza pandemic or other mass vaccination campaign.

Strategies

2.4.1
Expand collaboration with clinical, laboratory, genetic, statistical, and bioinformatics experts to conduct clinical research studies to investigate the role of host genetics in AEFIs.

2.4.2
Increase the size, representativeness, and utility of the population under active surveillance for serious AEFIs that can be included in timely, high quality, rigorously conducted epidemiological studies to assess vaccine safety questions.

Objective 2.5

Improve causality assessments of vaccines and related AEFIs.

Strategies

2.5.1
Build upon new scientific developments in areas such as genetics, systems biology and bioinformatics, and immunology to develop and validate tools which aid in (or enable) the identification of individual risk factors for AEFIs for which a causal relationship has been established.

2.5.2
Assess the evidence for a causal relationship between certain vaccines and specific clinically important AEFIs and, as the need arises, conduct an independent review of available evidence.

Objective 2.6

Improve scientific knowledge about why and among whom vaccine adverse reactions occur.

Strategies

2.6.1
Identify host risk factors that may be associated with increased risk for specific vaccine adverse reactions through basic, clinical, or epidemiological research.

2.6.2
Identify the biological mechanism(s) for vaccine adverse reactions.

2.6.3
Assess whether the risk of specific AEFIs is increased in specific populations such as pregnant women, premature infants, older adults, those with immunocompromising or other medical conditions, based on gender or race/ethnicity, or other at-risk individuals.

2.6.4
Develop a robust system to enhance collection of medical histories and biological specimens from selected persons experiencing serious AEFIs to enhance study of biological mechanisms and individual risk factors.

Objective 2.7

Improve clinical practice to prevent, identify and manage vaccine adverse reactions.

Strategies

2.7.1

Improve training, availability of, and access to vaccine safety clinical and communication experts to provide consultation to health care providers and public health practitioners.

2.7.2

Develop and disseminate evidence-based guidelines for vaccination or revaccination, as appropriate, especially for persons who may be at increased risk for vaccine adverse events. Use this information to clarify contraindications and precautions to vaccination.

Objective 2.8

Enhance collaboration of vaccine safety activities.

Strategies

2.8.1

Improve collaboration, such as data sharing arrangements, across federal agencies, departments, and with non-federal partners.

2.8.2

Improve information and data sharing with international partners (e.g., national vaccine safety programs) consistent with ethical and human subjects protections and applicable law, including confidentiality protections.

2.8.3

Develop additional standard case definitions for AEFIs for use in immunization safety surveillance and research, vaccine safety standards such as concept definitions, standardized abbreviations, and standardized study designs.

Goal 3:
Support communications to enhance informed vaccine decision-making

Introduction

HHS is committed to providing accurate, timely, transparent, complete, and audience-appropriate information about immunizations and vaccines. This information is designed for parents making vaccination decisions for their children (birth through age 18); adults considering vaccines for themselves; public health partners; providers; policy-makers and others.

Communication tools and channels used to disseminate immunization and vaccine information span a broad spectrum: publication of evidence-based recommendations; use of mass media and new media; provider education and training; and support of partner organizations and state immunization programs through provision of resources, trainings, updates, and announcements.

Current communication efforts are informed by research as well as the principles of effective risk communication, social marketing, and social mobilization. Research should be enhanced to better understand the nature of informed decision-making and the elements that support such decisions. Improved communications research can facilitate development of more targeted messages and methods for clearly and effectively communicating about the benefits and risks of vaccines, and to address information needs unique to various audiences. The combined efforts of communication scientists, health services researchers, and others can enhance the development and implementation of long-term, sustainable plans for gathering reliable real-time data about facilitators of and barriers to vaccine acceptance, translating those data into practical solutions. This research also enhances efforts to promote the adoption of vaccine recommendations to prevent disease and improve the public's health.

The 2010 National Vaccine Plan recognizes the importance of communication activities that are strategic, science-based, transparent, and culturally appropriate. Communication strategies should reflect the health literacy level and English proficiency of specific target population groups, as well as considerations of the accessibility of information to individuals with hearing, visual, cognitive, or other limitations. Related to these goals are the roles and responsibilities of various stakeholders engaged in vaccine communications and education. Policy-makers, such as federal, state, and local legislators; health departments; employers; third-party payors and others, are critical stakeholders in the vaccine enterprise. Collaborating with public health decision makers across the health sector is critical to realizing the full vision of the plan. Health care providers, advocacy groups, the public health community, and community and faith-based organizations can serve as strong and credible immunization advocates about the risk of VPDs, the benefits of vaccination, recommended schedules, the supply and financing of vaccines, and the possible risks associated with vaccination. Public-private collaboration on communication and education activities will be critical to achieving the goal and objectives set forth by the Plan.

While the focus of Goal 3 is on communication and education issues relevant to informed decision-making, these issues are also relevant to each of the other goals of the 2010 National Vaccine Plan. Topic-specific communications and education activities are described in Goals 2, 4, and 5.

Objectives

Objective 3.1
Utilize communication approaches that are based on ongoing research.

Strategies
3.1.1
Conduct research regularly to understand the public's knowledge, beliefs, and concerns about vaccines and VPDs.

3.1.2
Conduct research on factors that affect decision-making about vaccination for individuals and families, providers, and policy-makers.

3.1.3
Identify, develop, and test educational strategies that better enable policy-makers to read, understand, and use information about vaccine benefits and risks.

3.1.4
Evaluate the effectiveness of messages and materials in addressing the information needs and concerns of the public and under-immunized populations.

3.1.5
Develop evidence-based tools to assist individuals, parents, and providers with relevant information to make informed decisions regarding vaccination.

Objective 3.2:
Build and enhance collaborations and partnerships for communication efforts.

Strategies
3.2.1
Strengthen existing partnerships and coalitions and build relationships with new partners to support relevant immunizations across the lifespan.

3.2.2
Use cross-agency and intra-agency collaboration to inform development of communication research agendas, protocols, campaigns and messages.

3.2.3
Collaborate with partners and stakeholders to communicate vaccine benefits, risks, and recommendations in accessible formats and in culturally appropriate languages, methods, and literacy levels.

3.2.4
Utilize state and local venues to educate on vaccine and immunization issues to expand the reach of messages outside of the traditional clinical setting.

Objective 3.3

Enhance delivery of timely, accurate, and transparent information to public audiences and key intermediaries (such as media, providers, and public health officials) about what is known and unknown about the benefits and risks of vaccines.

Strategies

3.3.1

Enhance communication of new findings about vaccine effectiveness, safety, and administration studies to the public, partners and providers in a clear, transparent and timely manner.

3.3.2

Respond in a rapid, coordinated, consistent, and effective manner to emerging vaccine issues and concerns (e.g., supply, safety, or public health emergencies).

3.3.3

Rapidly and effectively disseminate communications research findings through peer-reviewed journals, conferences, media, and partner communications to facilitate implementation of evidence-based strategies.

Objective 3.4

Increase public awareness of the benefits and risks of vaccines and immunization, especially among populations at risk of under-immunization.

Strategies

3.4.1

Develop, implement, and evaluate a long-term strategic communications plan and program aimed at educating parents, caregivers of children, adolescents, and adults about VPDs; the benefits and risks of vaccines; and vaccine recommendations.

3.4.2

Maintain current, easily accessible, evidence-based online information on VPDs and vaccines, including benefits and risks and the basis of immunization recommendations, for all audience groups.

3.4.3

Evaluate new media (such as mobile technologies and social media) and utilize it appropriately to reach target audiences with accurate and timely information about vaccines and to respond to emerging concerns and issues.

3.4.4

Enhance awareness of the importance of immunization as part of preventive health care among parents, adolescents, and adults.

3.4.5

Collaborate with the education community to assess opportunities to integrate information on VPDs, recommended vaccines, preventive health care, and public health in existing educational curricula.

3.4.6

Develop and disseminate vaccine communication tools/materials that are accessible and culturally and literacy-level appropriate for groups at risk of under-immunization.

Objective 3.5:

Assure that key decision- and policy-makers (e.g., third-party payers, employers, legislators, community leaders, hospital administrators, health departments) receive accurate and timely information on vaccine benefits and risks; economics; and public and stakeholder knowledge, attitudes, and beliefs.

Strategies

3.5.1

Develop, disseminate, and evaluate broad-based education tools for key groups on the value, risks, and cost-effectiveness of vaccines; the basis of immunization recommendations; business case evidence and guidance; vaccine policy development; the standards of immunization practice and administration; and vaccines as a component of preventive health care.

3.5.2

Select and implement a model for sustained community engagement to inform vaccine policy and program activities.

3.5.3

Provide vaccine program managers and policy-makers information on the direct and indirect costs and benefits of vaccination. This includes, but is not limited to, information on federal and state programs that offer low-cost vaccines.

3.5.4

Provide policy-makers with data necessary to make informed decisions on the utilization of vaccines in mass vaccination programs for public health emergencies.

Goal 4:

Ensure a stable supply of, access to, and better use of recommended vaccines in the United States

Introduction

VPD incidence in the U.S. is at or near record-low levels for most diseases against which children are routinely immunized; infant and child vaccination rates are approaching or meet record levels. However, coverage levels are below HP 2020 targets for many vaccines targeted to adolescents and adults, and substantial disparities exist among racial and ethnic groups in adult and adolescent vaccination levels. Limited knowledge about recommended vaccines and attitudes towards vaccines exist among the public, health care professionals, and health policy- and decision-makers. Lack of health care access and financial barriers also contribute to these disparities and need to be addressed in strategies moving forward. Research on how best to overcome such barriers will dictate strategies and practices. Ongoing partnerships among national, state, local, tribal, private, and public entities are needed to sustain and improve vaccine use and the concomitant individual and public health benefits.

Ensuring a reliable and steady supply of all vaccines is critical in the U.S., where shortages of several commonly used vaccines have occurred since 2000 (e.g., Hib, hepatitis A, and influenza). New 21st-century vaccine supply concerns, such as vaccines for pandemic influenza, emerging diseases and bioterrorism threats, present different challenges for sustainability and may require surge manufacturing capacity compared with traditional vaccine pathways.

Immunization information systems (IIS) and electronic health records (EHR) may become increasingly important components of immunization programs. Jointly they can lead to much better immunization recordkeeping for children and adults, thereby reducing the barrier of unknown immunization status and the receipt of additional unneeded doses of vaccines and enhancing efficiency and cost-effectiveness of national immunization efforts.

Strong public health surveillance to monitor and evaluate VPDs and the effectiveness of licensed vaccines provides the link between vaccination policy and health outcomes. Such public health surveillance is a key component of strategies to overcome barriers and improve use of existing vaccines.

Challenges persist to improve vaccination rates and to incorporate new vaccines into child and adolescent vaccination schedules. Between 2005 and 2010, six new vaccines or vaccine recommendations were added for children and adolescents by the ACIP and the Centers for Disease Control and Prevention (CDC):

- meningococcal conjugate vaccine

- tetanus, diphtheria, acellular pertussis vaccine

- HPV vaccine

- rotavirus vaccine

- universal influenza vaccination

- 13-valent pneumococcal conjugate vaccine.

Barriers to improved vaccine uptake include persistent cost, awareness and access problems; lack of knowledge of necessary vaccines; and limited use of evidence-based strategies to improve vaccine uptake, such as reminder-recall systems. Community health centers, other community immunization sites (e.g., pharmacies and stores) and school-located clinics offer venues for improving vaccine uptake, in addition to traditional provider sites.

Goal 4 identifies nine objectives and related strategies to strengthen our nation's vaccination program and overcome barriers. Enhancing communication and education activities about vaccination is a key approach to overcome many of the current challenges identified in Goal 4, and is addressed in detail in Goal 3.

Objectives

Objective 4.1
Ensure consistent and adequate supply of vaccines for the U.S.

Strategies
4.1.1
Determine barriers to having multiple suppliers for each vaccine licensed and recommended for routine use in the U.S.

4.1.2
Promote harmonization of international vaccine regulatory standards for licensure.

4.1.3
Improve vaccine quality and availability through better manufacturing and production oversight.

4.1.4
Optimize use, content, and distribution of vaccine stockpiles and ancillary supplies.

4.1.5
Improve the development of, communication of, and tracking of adherence to recommended changes in vaccine use during national vaccine shortages.

Objective 4.2
Ensure consistent and stable delivery of vaccines for the U.S.

Strategies
4.2.1
Improve vaccine ordering, distribution and tracking systems for routine use, for public health emergencies, and for management of delivery disruptions.

4.2.2
Enhance public sector infrastructure to support and sustain adult immunization activities, including addressing disparities in vaccination rates among racial and ethnic minorities and unvaccinated refugees resettling to the U.S.

4.2.3
Expand access to vaccination at medical care sites for children, adolescents, and adults, such as by increasing hours of operation and establishing specific vaccination clinics at selected times of the year (e.g., "back to school" campaigns).

4.2.4
Expand access to vaccination in non-health care settings, such as retail outlets, schools, workplaces, and community centers.

4.2.5
Develop, monitor, and evaluate policies promoting vaccination for patients in long-term care facilities and hospitals.

4.2.6
Develop, implement, and evaluate employer-based immunization programs, which should include free vaccines, convenient access, education, and compliance monitoring, to increase the coverage of employees, including health care workers, with recommended vaccines.

4.2.7
Implement, monitor, and evaluate evidence-based interventions designed to raise and sustain high vaccination coverage across the lifespan.

4.2.8
Monitor and evaluate the impact of state immunization laws and regulations on vaccine coverage, including childcare, pre-school, school, college prematriculation requirements, employer requirements, and the role of exemptions, insurance mandates, and immunization information systems requirements.

4.2.9
Prepare, practice, and evaluate mass vaccination activities, including vaccine administration, for scenarios such as an outbreak of a VPD, for a biological attack, for the critical workforce in advance of an influenza pandemic, and for the entire population, prior to and during, an influenza pandemic.

Objective 4.3
Reduce financial barriers to vaccination.

Strategies
4.3.1
Identify and regularly monitor financial barriers to receipt of ACIP-recommended and CDC-adopted vaccines.

4.3.2
Ensure that out-of-pocket costs for purchase and administration of ACIP-recommended and CDC-adopted vaccines do not represent a significant financial barrier.

4.3.3
Strengthen the ability of states to purchase, and expand access to, ACIP-recommended and CDC-adopted vaccines for those who qualify for publicly supported vaccinations.

4.3.4
Develop, implement, and evaluate strategies to reduce the financial burden on vaccination providers for purchase of initial and ongoing vaccine inventories.

Objective 4.4

Maintain and enhance the capacity to monitor immunization coverage for vaccines routinely administered to all age groups.

Strategies

4.4.1

Identify, implement, and evaluate cost-effective and rapid methods, such as the use of IIS or internet panel surveys, for assessing vaccination coverage by categories, including age groups, groups at risk of under immunization, by type of vaccine, and type of financing.

4.4.2

Improve the completeness of, use of, and communication between, IIS and EHR to monitor vaccination coverage.

4.4.3

Support the adoption of national certified, interoperable health information technology and EHR for immunization.

4.4.4

Support and improve existing surveys assessing immunization coverage (e.g., the National Immunization Survey and the Behavioral Risk Factor Surveillance System), to include more representative samples and timely reporting of data.

Objective 4.5

Enhance tracking of VPDs and monitoring of the effectiveness of licensed vaccines.

Strategies

4.5.1

Strengthen epidemiologic and laboratory methods and tools to diagnose VPDs, assess population susceptibility, and characterize vaccine effectiveness and the impact of vaccination coverage on clinical and public health outcomes.

4.5.2

Monitor circulating strains of relevant vaccine-preventable and potentially vaccine-preventable pathogens, including emerging and re-emerging diseases.

4.5.3

Improve monitoring of disease burden and determine epidemiologic and clinical characteristics of cases of VPDs and potential VPDs by supporting traditional surveillance and use of health information technology, interoperable data standards, and new data resources.

4.5.4

Develop and maintain capacity to rapidly estimate the effectiveness of new vaccines, such as pandemic and pre-pandemic influenza vaccines.

4.5.5

Assure rapid and comprehensive identification, investigation, and response to vaccine-preventable disease outbreaks.

4.5.6
Assure timely evaluation to assess vaccine effectiveness, duration of protection, and indirect (community and herd) protection by current and newly recommended vaccines.

Objective 4.6
Educate and support health care providers in vaccination counseling and vaccine delivery for their patients and themselves.

Strategies

4.6.1
Expand and implement training and education of health care providers on VPDs, including diagnosis, modes of transmission, prevention and control, and reporting requirements.

4.6.2
Expand and implement training and education of immunization providers at all levels of their education on the proper use and administration of vaccines; the proper storage and handling of vaccines; the basis of immunization recommendations; the safety of vaccines; reporting of AEFIs; understanding of the vaccine safety system; and on the standards of immunization practice (e.g., vaccine education modules in primary care and continuing medical education programs).

4.6.3
Develop a plan to reduce and ultimately eliminate errors in vaccine administration (e.g., wrong vaccine, dose, injection site, or timing).

4.6.4
Promote and support educational and technical assistance to improve business practices associated with providing immunizations, such as educating providers and enrolling new providers into the Vaccines for Children program, including non-traditional providers.

4.6.5
Expand the incorporation of vaccinations and the use of IIS into quality improvement programs such as the Healthcare Effectiveness Data and Information Set.

4.6.6
Support adequate reimbursement for vaccine counseling, administration, storage and handling by providers under public sector and private health plans.

4.6.7
Support research to evaluate the capacity (accommodating the increased number of patient visits required to receive recommended vaccines) of health care providers to implement vaccine recommendations for all age groups.

4.6.8
Develop, implement, and evaluate comprehensive programs to ensure health care professionals are appropriately immunized with recommended vaccines.

Objective 4.7

Maintain a strong, science-based, transparent process for developing and evaluating immunization recommendations.

Strategies

4.7.1

Obtain broad-based input from the public and stakeholders contributing to new immunization policies and the assessment of existing policies.

4.7.2

Assess the impact of new vaccines and vaccine recommendations on the overall immunization schedule, including programmatic implementation, safety, and efficacy.

4.7.3

Evaluate the cost-effectiveness and comparative effectiveness of proposed and existing immunization recommendations.

Objective 4.8

Strengthen the National Vaccine Injury Compensation Program (VICP) and Countermeasures Injury Compensation Program (CICP).

Strategies

4.8.1

Increase knowledge about the VICP and CICP among all stakeholders.

4.8.2

Assure the programs are responsive to evolving science, including regularly updating their Vaccine Injury Tables.

4.8.3

Continue to ensure fair and efficient compensation for vaccine-related injuries.

4.8.4

Examine alternative approaches, and evaluate and implement those deemed optimal, for adjudication of VICP claims for illnesses not included in the Vaccine Injury Table to the extent permitted by applicable law.

Objective 4.9

Enhance immunization coverage for travelers.

Strategies

4.9.1

Define the populations at risk for acquiring international travel-related VPDs, and identify and address barriers to their receiving immunizations.

4.9.2

Assess overall immunization status during travel-related immunization clinics.

Goal 5:
Increase global prevention of death and disease through safe and effective vaccination

Introduction
Infectious diseases are the leading cause of death among children globally and contribute substantially to disease and disability among persons of all ages. Immunization programs have been remarkably successful in preventing millions of childhood deaths, eradicating smallpox, and eliminating circulation of polio and measles from many countries around the world. However, substantial challenges remain. Many diseases for which safe and effective vaccines are available pose a continued burden, as does the underutilization of vaccines in most countries (e.g., pneumococcal, rotavirus and HPV) and diseases for which vaccines are being developed (e.g., HIV, TB, and malaria). Globally mobile populations including refugees, and stateless and internally displaced persons are often difficult to reach and may not be included in national immunization programs. Achieving the United Nations' Millennium Development Goals of reducing the under-five year mortality rate by two thirds by 2015 will require substantive action, including increasing the proportion of one year-old children immunized against measles.

The goals of global vaccination are to control, eliminate, or eradicate infectious diseases in a way that strengthens health systems and is sustainable as new vaccines are introduced. Success in global immunization requires action by the full range of stakeholders involved in the vaccine and immunization enterprise: research and development, regulation and manufacturing, and program implementation and monitoring. New partnerships such as the Global Alliance for Vaccines and Immunizations (GAVI) have led to increased support for immunization worldwide, spurring introduction of new vaccines in low income countries and expanded vaccination coverage. U.S. governmental and NGOs have contributed to progress through vaccine research and development, participation in multilateral and bilateral partnerships, technical assistance, and program support.

Given the breadth of global immunization activities in Goal 5, some of the objectives and strategies relevant to this topic are included elsewhere in this Plan. For example, all vaccine research and development issues are included under Goal 1 because the approach and stakeholders necessary to achieve these objectives are largely the same in the U.S. and the rest of the world. Similarly, issues related to vaccine safety, communications and program implementation are included under this goal, as well as under other goals of the Plan, as there are unique intellectual perspectives for them. While many of the objectives in these areas are similar for the U.S. and abroad, the strategies differ internationally because U.S. stakeholders focus on partnerships and providing assistance rather than on direct implementation.

In the era of global pandemics and mass travel, the public health of U.S. citizens is closely related to diseases occurring in other countries. Even though many VPDs such as polio, measles, and rubella have been eliminated in this country, the U.S. remains vulnerable to importations as long as these diseases continue to persist elsewhere. Support for overseas (pre-departure) vaccination of mobile populations, including refugees and immigrants migrating to the U.S., will reduce the likelihood of importation. Support for developing and introducing new vaccines to address diseases in other countries and assisting with strengthening and enhancing capacity of their immunization programs contributes toward providing an "umbrella of protection" for the U S. and fulfilling the U.S. government's broader commitment to global public health.

Meeting this commitment to support global immunization is also reflected in other federal public health initiatives and development initiatives beyond the Plan. The GHI – currently led by the U.S.

Department of State, USAID, and the CDC, with active engagement of other agencies, including the Department of Defense (DoD), NIH, and the Health Resources Services Administration (HRSA) – and FDA's global vaccine regulatory capacity building efforts through the World Health Organization (WHO) are two examples of federal initiatives that incorporate immunization as a component of a broad U.S. interest to improve maternal and child health. Additionally, the CDC has a Global Immunization Strategic Framework that focuses on how the agency will support immunization programs around the world. These and other initiatives are consistent with the objectives outlined in the Plan.

Objectives

Objective 5.1
Support international organizations and countries to improve global surveillance for VPDs and strengthen health information systems to monitor vaccine coverage, effectiveness, and safety.

Strategies
5.1.1
Achieve sustainable WHO certification quality surveillance for eradication of targeted VPDs.

5.1.2
Expand and improve sustainable surveillance systems for all diseases having WHO-recommended vaccines and diseases for which vaccine introduction is being considered.

5.1.3
Strengthen all levels of global laboratory networks (including national, regional, and global reference laboratories) to sustain and improve VPD diagnosis in order to establish baseline disease burden, detect outbreaks, detect newly emerging variants of VPDs, and monitor the impact of new vaccines. This laboratory capacity should also be developed for surveillance of potential public health emergencies of international concern.

5.1.4
Enhance assessments of emerging variants or strains of VPD agents.

5.1.5
Develop new diagnostic tests, tools and procedures to improve both field-based and laboratory confirmation of diagnoses.

Objective 5.2
Support international organizations and countries to improve and sustain immunization programs as a component of health care delivery systems and promote opportunities to link immunization delivery with other priority health interventions, where appropriate.

Strategies
5.2.1
Provide technical support to countries, multilateral institutions, and other partners to strengthen key components of immunization program management and implementation, including epidemiological analysis, comprehensive planning, vaccine distribution and safe administration, monitoring, information systems, and program evaluation.

5.2.2
Provide technical support to countries and multilateral institutions as appropriate to introduce, sustain, and monitor recommended safe injection practices for all vaccinations, including the use of auto disable syringes or needle-free devices.

5.2.3
Improve coverage monitoring of vaccines and other health services linked with the vaccination program and the use of information at district and local levels.

5.2.4
Introduce and improve programs that evaluate AEFIs.

5.2.5
Develop standardized methods for monitoring and evaluating the efficiency, effectiveness and impact of combined interventions to improve coverage, and support linking delivery of immunization and other health services in ways that do not jeopardize immunization coverage.

5.2.6
Encourage establishment of programs, as appropriate, for vaccination beyond the traditional infant target age groups (e.g., among older children, adolescents, adults, and health care providers), including unvaccinated mobile populations of various age groups since the epidemiology in some mobile populations may differ from other populations where the diseases are normally spreading in certain age-groups.

5.2.7
Provide technical support to countries, multilateral institutions as appropriate, and other partners to develop sustainable vaccine financing mechanisms and adequate global supplies of vaccines, including through economic and supply and demand analyses.

Objective 5.3
Support international organizations and countries to introduce and make available new and underutilized vaccines to prevent diseases of public health importance.

Strategies
5.3.1
Strengthen capacity at the country level, and in multilateral institutions as appropriate, to make informed decisions on introduction of new vaccines based on evaluation of epidemiology, financial sustainability, safety, and programmatic considerations, including support to national advisory committees.

5.3.2
Collaborate with global organizations and partners to accelerate clinical testing and licensure in developing countries of vaccines already licensed in developed countries, where appropriate.

5.3.3
Support the integration of new and underutilized vaccines into each GAVI-eligible country's multi-year national plan of action and provide training and logistical support necessary to successfully incorporate new vaccines into routine programs.

5.3.4
Support post-licensure evaluations of new vaccines with regard to immunization programs, disease patterns, and vaccine safety.

5.3.5
Work with global partners to establish an international system that facilitates rapid response to emerging infections through the development of vaccine reference strains and candidate vaccines.

5.3.6
Work with global partners to secure and maintain adequate stockpiles/strategic reserves of vaccines to maintain uninterrupted supply and for emergency response to outbreaks.

5.3.7
Support and develop mechanisms for rapidly making vaccines available to developing countries for public health emergencies such as pandemic influenza, including exploring options for sharing of vaccines and tiered pricing.

Objective 5.4
Support international organizations and countries to improve communication of evidence-based and culturally and linguistically appropriate information about the benefits and risks of vaccines to the public, providers, and policy-makers.

Strategies
5.4.1
Support appropriate economic studies to inform key decision- and policy-makers' understanding of the benefits and costs of immunization.

5.4.2
Support the development of capabilities to communicate vaccine benefits and risks and to respond to emerging vaccine safety issues.

5.4.3
Support national systems to improve reporting of adverse events.

5.4.4
Assist countries to develop and implement sustainable communication research to gather timely and reliable data from the public and providers on knowledge, attitudes and beliefs about the benefits and risks of vaccines.

5.4.5
Assist countries to develop communication plans to increase provider and public awareness of VPDs and promote immunization recommendations, especially among populations at risk of under-immunization.

5.4.6
Provide technical assistance and training to behavioral and communications scientists and promote their participation on Technical Advisory Groups.

5.4.7
Support and participate with partners to create and implement a global vaccine advocacy strategy.

Objective 5.5

Support the development of regulatory environments and manufacturing capabilities that facilitate access to safe and effective vaccines in all countries.

Strategies

5.5.1

Promote and support the efforts of WHO and other global partners to develop and harmonize international standards for vaccine development and licensure.

5.5.2

Promote and support the efforts of WHO and others to improve regulatory capacity in countries with limited infrastructures to assure vaccine quality, evaluate new vaccines when appropriate, and assure that clinical trials are conducted in accordance with Good Clinical Practices.

5.5.3

Provide technical assistance to developing country vaccine manufacturers to support development and production of safe and effective vaccines.

Objective 5.6

Build and strengthen multilateral and bilateral partnerships and other collaborative efforts to support global immunization and eradication programs.

Strategies

5.6.1

Participate in establishing global immunization priorities, goals and objectives and provide technical assistance at global, regional, and national levels.

5.6.2

Strengthen international collaborations for basic and applied research and related training of next generation researchers, especially in disease endemic areas, to include improving the stability and performance of current vaccines.

5.6.3

Contribute to development and implementation of a plan establishing the scientific basis for VPD eradication/elimination, identifying optimal vaccination approaches, and developing strategies to minimize risks in the post-eradication period.

5.6.4

Participate in regional immunization initiatives, such as those adopted by the Pan American Health Organization and other WHO regions.

5.6.5

Strengthen vaccination of globally mobile populations through targeted programs (e.g., pre-departure vaccination of US bound refugees).

Monitoring and Evaluation

NVPO will be responsible for assuring coordination and for monitoring federal actions and accomplishments on the 2010 National Vaccine Plan on an ongoing basis. NVPO and NVAC will report their findings to the Assistant Secretary for Health annually. This report will include a summary of progress, identify areas where progress is lagging, and propose corrective action where needed. The report also will be presented at an NVAC meeting, which is open to the public and is attended by many stakeholders not represented directly on the Committee.

Key federal stakeholders in global immunization include CDC, the Department of State and USAID. Many of the global immunization targets included in the Plan were established by international organizations (e.g., WHO) in consultation with U.S. stakeholders. However, the role of those stakeholders in achieving these targets most often involves providing technical assistance and support rather than direct implementation.

Many factors may affect the ability to achieve National Vaccine Plan objectives. Opportunities may emerge that facilitate rapid progress and achievement of objectives sooner than anticipated. Scientific, technological, health care financing, or communications advances also could emerge and enable rapid achievement of the vision laid forth by the Plan, superseding its objectives and goals. On the other hand, existing challenges and barriers may be more difficult to overcome than anticipated and new challenges may emerge. For example, a range of scientific and technical issues may delay development and licensure of new vaccines; safety concerns may affect vaccine uptake; financial constraints may affect vaccination delivery. Recognizing these uncertainties, NVPO will coordinate a mid-course review of the Plan after five years allowing changes to be made which respond to the reality of the environment. Modified indicators, strategies, actions, and milestones will guide subsequent annual evaluation through the overall ten-year horizon of the Plan.

Conclusion

The overriding goal of this plan is to invigorate national coordination and planning on vaccines and immunizations. HHS will lead this national effort, leveraging existing resources and expertise, to maximize the control of VPDs in this country and with global partners. Given that this is intended to be not just a federal plan but represent a national strategy, it will require the partnership of stakeholders involved in all aspects of the vaccine enterprise. The goals, objectives, and strategies outlined in this document, when fully implemented, will markedly enhance the control of VPDs and the health of the public in this nation.

Table 2:
National Vaccine Plan Objectives: Responsible Stakeholders

Objective				Federal													
				HHS													
	ACF	AHRQ	ASPR (BARDA)	CDC	CMS	FDA	HRSA	IHS	NIH	NVPO	ONC	DHS	DoD	DoJ	Dept. of State	USAID	VA
Goal 1: Develop new and improved vaccines																	
1.1			✓	✓		✓		✓	✓	✓			✓			✓	✓
1.2			✓	✓		✓				✓			✓			✓	✓
1.3			✓	✓						✓			✓			✓	✓
1.4			✓			✓				✓			✓				✓
1.5		✓							✓	✓		✓	✓			✓	
1.6			✓			✓				✓			✓				✓
Goal 2: Enhance the vaccine safety system																	
2.1			✓			✓	✓		✓	✓			✓				✓
2.2						✓							✓				
2.3			✓	✓	✓	✓	✓			✓			✓				✓
2.4		✓	✓	✓	✓	✓	✓			✓			✓				✓
2.5			✓	✓	✓	✓	✓			✓			✓				✓
2.6			✓			✓	✓	✓	✓				✓				✓
2.7			✓	✓		✓		✓		✓			✓				✓
2.8		✓	✓	✓	✓	✓	✓			✓			✓			✓	✓
Goal 3: Support communications to enhance informed vaccine decision-making																	
3.1	✓		✓	✓	✓	✓		✓	✓	✓			✓				✓
3.2	✓		✓	✓	✓	✓	✓	✓	✓	✓			✓				✓
3.3	✓		✓	✓	✓	✓	✓	✓	✓	✓			✓				✓
3.4	✓		✓	✓	✓	✓	✓	✓	✓	✓			✓				✓
3.5	✓		✓	✓	✓	✓	✓	✓	✓	✓			✓				✓
Goal 4: Ensure a stable supply of, access to and better use of recommended vaccines in the United States																	
4.1			✓	✓		✓	✓	✓		✓			✓				✓
4.2			✓	✓		✓	✓	✓					✓			✓	✓
4.3			✓	✓				✓								✓	✓
4.4			✓	✓		✓	✓				✓		✓				
4.5			✓	✓		✓	✓	✓	✓				✓			✓	✓
4.6		✓	✓	✓	✓	✓	✓	✓		✓			✓			✓	✓
4.7		✓	✓			✓	✓	✓		✓							
4.8	✓		✓	✓			✓	✓				✓	✓	✓			✓
4.9	✓		✓										✓		✓	✓	✓
Goal 5: Increase global prevention of death and disease through safe and effective vaccination																	
5.1			✓						✓				✓		✓	✓	
5.2			✓										✓		✓	✓	
5.3			✓			✓			✓						✓	✓	
5.4			✓												✓	✓	
5.5		✓	✓			✓									✓	✓	
5.6			✓			✓			✓				✓		✓	✓	

Department of Health & Human Services | The 2010 National Vaccine Plan

Objective	Non-federal									
	Health care providers	Health care system	Public and private health care plans	State, local, and tribal governments	Academia	Advocacy organizations	Philanthropic organizations	Vaccine manufacturers	UNICEF	WHO
Goal 1: Develop new and improved vaccines										
1.1	✓			✓	✓		✓	✓		✓
1.2					✓		✓	✓		
1.3					✓		✓	✓		
1.4					✓		✓	✓		
1.5					✓		✓	✓		
1.6					✓			✓		
Goal 2: Enhance the vaccine safety system										
2.1				✓	✓	✓		✓		
2.2					✓			✓		
2.3		✓	✓	✓	✓			✓		
2.4		✓	✓	✓	✓			✓		
2.5		✓	✓	✓	✓			✓		
2.6					✓			✓		
2.7		✓	✓	✓	✓			✓		
2.8		✓			✓			✓		✓
Goal 3: Support communications to enhance informed vaccine decision-making										
3.1		✓	✓	✓	✓			✓		
3.2	✓	✓	✓	✓	✓	✓		✓		
3.3	✓	✓	✓	✓	✓	✓		✓		
3.4	✓	✓	✓	✓		✓		✓		
3.5		✓	✓	✓	✓	✓		✓		
Goal 4: Ensure a stable supply of, access to and better use of recommended vaccines in the United States										
4.1	✓	✓	✓	✓				✓		
4.2	✓	✓	✓	✓				✓		
4.3		✓	✓	✓						
4.4	✓	✓	✓	✓	✓	✓	✓	✓		
4.5		✓	✓	✓			✓	✓		
4.6	✓	✓		✓		✓		✓		
4.7		✓		✓		✓		✓		
4.8		✓		✓		✓	✓	✓		
4.9	✓	✓	✓	✓				✓		
Goal 5: Increase global prevention of death and disease through safe and effective vaccination										
5.1					✓	✓	✓		✓	✓
5.2					✓	✓	✓		✓	✓
5.3					✓	✓	✓		✓	✓
5.4					✓	✓	✓		✓	✓
5.5					✓	✓	✓	✓		✓
5.6					✓	✓	✓		✓	✓